PLANT-BASED LUPUS COOKBOOK
FOR WOMEN

Anti-Inflammatory Recipes to Support Lupus Management and Promote Overall Wellness

Over **100** Healing recipes

JUDY KELLY

Copyright © Judy Kelly, 2024.

Table of Contents

Introduction

Welcome to a journey of health and healing through the power of plant-based nutrition. This cookbook is dedicated to all the women who face the daily challenges of living with lupus, a chronic autoimmune disease that can affect every aspect of life.

Living with lupus requires not just physical resilience, but also emotional strength and unwavering determination. It's a journey of ups and downs, of victories and setbacks. But through it all, one thing remains constant – the power of nourishing our bodies with wholesome, plant-based foods.

This cookbook is not just a collection of recipes; it's a testament to the resilience and courage of women with lupus. It's a celebration of the strength that comes from taking charge of our health and embracing a lifestyle that supports our well-being.

In these pages, you'll find a variety of delicious and nutrient-rich recipes designed to support your health and vitality. Each recipe is crafted with care, keeping in mind the unique challenges that lupus presents. From hearty breakfasts to satisfying dinners, from refreshing drinks to indulgent desserts – there's something here for every meal and every craving.

But more than just recipes, this cookbook is a companion on your journey to better health. It's a reminder that you're not alone – that there's a community of women just like you, striving every day to live their best lives despite lupus.

So, as you embark on this culinary adventure, I invite you to savor not just the flavors of these dishes, but also the joy of nourishing your body and soul. Here's to health, here's to strength, and here's to you, amazing women with lupus.

About This Cookbook

Welcome to the "Plant-Based Lupus Cookbook for Women" – a resource designed to empower women living with lupus to embrace a healthier lifestyle through plant-based nutrition.

Our Mission

At the heart of this cookbook is a simple yet powerful mission: to provide women with lupus the tools they need to take control of their health and well-being. We believe that food is medicine, and that the right nutrition can play a crucial role in managing lupus symptoms and improving overall quality of life.

What Sets This Cookbook Apart

This cookbook is more than just a collection of recipes. It's a comprehensive guide to navigating the challenges of living with lupus while embracing a plant-based diet. Here's what sets it apart:

1. Expert Guidance: Each recipe in this cookbook is carefully crafted with input from nutrition experts and healthcare professionals who specialize in autoimmune diseases like lupus. You can trust that these recipes are not only delicious but also designed to support your health.

2. Tailored for Women: Recognizing that lupus affects women differently than men, this cookbook is specifically tailored to address the unique nutritional needs and challenges faced by women with lupus.

3. Accessible Ingredients: You won't find any obscure or hard-to-find ingredients in these recipes. We've made sure that all the ingredients are readily available at your local grocery store, making it easy to whip up nutritious meals without hassle.

4. Variety and Flexibility: Whether you're a seasoned cook or just starting out on your plant-based journey, you'll find something here to suit your tastes and preferences. From quick and easy weeknight dinners to elegant dishes for special occasions, there's something for every occasion and every palate.

How to Use This Cookbook

- Explore: Take some time to browse through the recipes and familiarize yourself with the ingredients and instructions.
- Plan: Use the meal planning tips and suggestions provided to create a balanced and nutritious meal plan that works for you.
- Cook: Roll up your sleeves, gather your ingredients, and get cooking! Don't be afraid to experiment and make these recipes your own.
- Enjoy: Sit back, relax, and savor the delicious flavors of your plant-based creations. And remember, every meal you enjoy from this cookbook is a step towards better health and well-being.

Thank you for choosing this cookbook to accompany you on your journey to a healthier, happier life with lupus.

Understanding Lupus and Diet

Lupus is a complex autoimmune disease that can affect multiple systems in the body, including the joints, skin, kidneys, heart, and brain. While there is no cure for lupus, managing the condition often involves a combination of medication, lifestyle changes, and dietary modifications.

The Role of Diet in Lupus Management

Diet can play a significant role in managing lupus symptoms and improving overall health and well-being. While there is no one-size-fits-all diet for lupus, making certain dietary changes can help alleviate symptoms and improve quality of life.

Anti-Inflammatory Foods

Inflammation is a key driver of lupus symptoms, so focusing on an anti-inflammatory diet can be beneficial. This includes incorporating plenty of fruits, vegetables, whole grains, and healthy fats into your meals. Foods rich in antioxidants, such as berries, leafy greens, and nuts, can help reduce inflammation and protect against damage caused by free radicals.

Omega-3 Fatty Acids

Omega-3 fatty acids, found in fatty fish like salmon, sardines, and mackerel, as well as in flaxseeds, chia seeds, and walnuts, have been shown to have anti-inflammatory properties. Including these foods in your diet can help reduce inflammation and improve symptoms of lupus.

Limiting Trigger Foods

Some people with lupus find that certain foods can trigger or worsen their symptoms. Common trigger foods include processed foods, refined sugars, and saturated fats. Keeping a food diary can help you identify any foods that may be exacerbating your symptoms, allowing you to make more informed dietary choices.

Benefits of a Plant-Based Diet for Women with Lupus

A plant-based diet, which focuses on whole, minimally processed plant foods, has been shown to offer several benefits for women with lupus. While individual responses to diet can vary, many women with lupus find that adopting a plant-based diet can help improve their symptoms and overall quality of life.

Reduced Inflammation

One of the key benefits of a plant-based diet for women with lupus is its ability to reduce inflammation in the body. Plant foods are rich in antioxidants and phytonutrients, which can help combat inflammation and reduce the severity of lupus symptoms.

Improved Gut Health

A plant-based diet can also help improve gut health, which is important for women with lupus. A healthy gut microbiome is crucial for a strong immune system and can help reduce inflammation throughout the body.

Weight Management

Maintaining a healthy weight is important for women with lupus, as excess weight can put added strain on the joints and exacerbate symptoms. A plant-based diet, which is typically lower in calories and saturated fats than a standard Western diet, can help women with lupus manage their weight more effectively.

Heart Health

Heart disease is a common complication of lupus, so maintaining heart health is crucial. A plant-based diet has been shown to lower cholesterol levels, reduce blood pressure, and improve overall heart health, which can benefit women with lupus.

While a plant-based diet may not be a cure for lupus, many women find that it can help improve their symptoms and quality of life. By focusing on whole, nutrient-rich plant foods, women with lupus can support their overall health and well-being and better manage their condition.

Chapter 1: Breakfast Recipes

1. QUINOA BREAKFAST BOWL

Ingredients:
- 1/2 cup quinoa, rinsed
- 1 cup almond milk (or your choice of plant-based milk)
- 1 tablespoon maple syrup
- 1/2 teaspoon ground cinnamon
- 1/4 cup chopped nuts (such as almonds, walnuts, or pecans)
- Fresh berries, for topping
- Fresh mint leaves, for garnish

Instructions:
1. In a medium saucepan, combine the quinoa, almond milk, maple syrup, and cinnamon. Bring to a boil, then reduce heat and simmer, covered, for 15-20 minutes, or until the quinoa is tender and the liquid is absorbed.
2. Remove from heat and let sit, covered, for 5 minutes. Fluff with a fork.
3. Serve the quinoa in bowls, topped with chopped nuts, fresh berries, and a few mint leaves for garnish.

2. CHIA SEED PUDDING

Ingredients:
- 1/4 cup chia seeds
- 1 cup almond milk (or your choice of plant-based milk)
- 1 tablespoon maple syrup
- 1/2 teaspoon vanilla extract
- Fresh fruit, for topping
- Unsweetened coconut flakes, for garnish

Instructions:
1. In a bowl, combine the chia seeds, almond milk, maple syrup, and vanilla extract. Stir well to combine.

2. Cover and refrigerate for at least 2 hours, or overnight, until the mixture thickens and becomes pudding-like.
3. Serve the chia seed pudding in bowls, topped with fresh fruit and a sprinkle of unsweetened coconut flakes.

3. BLUEBERRY OATMEAL

Ingredients:
- 1/2 cup rolled oats
- 1 cup water
- 1/2 cup blueberries (fresh or frozen)
- 1 tablespoon almond butter
- 1 tablespoon maple syrup
- Pinch of cinnamon

Instructions:
1. In a small saucepan, bring the water to a boil. Stir in the oats and reduce heat to low. Cook, stirring occasionally, for 5-7 minutes, or until the oats are tender and creamy.
2. Stir in the blueberries, almond butter, maple syrup, and cinnamon. Cook for an additional 2-3 minutes, or until the blueberries are heated through.
3. Serve the oatmeal in bowls, topped with additional blueberries and a drizzle of maple syrup if desired.

4. AVOCADO TOAST WITH TOMATOES

Ingredients:
- 2 slices whole grain bread
- 1 ripe avocado
- 1 small tomato, sliced
- Salt and pepper, to taste
- Red pepper flakes, for garnish (optional)
- Fresh basil leaves, for garnish (optional)

Instructions:
1. Toast the bread to your desired level of crispiness.
2. While the bread is toasting, mash the avocado in a bowl with a fork until smooth.
3. Spread the mashed avocado evenly onto the toasted bread slices.
4. Top each slice with tomato slices, and season with salt, pepper, red pepper flakes, and fresh basil leaves if desired.

5. SMOOTHIE BOWL

Ingredients:
- 1 frozen banana
- 1/2 cup frozen mixed berries
- 1/2 cup spinach leaves
- 1/2 cup almond milk (or your choice of plant-based milk)
- Toppings: granola, sliced bananas, berries, chia seeds, shredded coconut

Instructions:
1. In a blender, combine the frozen banana, frozen mixed berries, spinach, and almond milk. Blend until smooth.
2. Pour the smoothie into a bowl and top with granola, sliced bananas, berries, chia seeds, and shredded coconut.

6. TURMERIC GINGER OATMEAL

Ingredients:
- 1/2 cup rolled oats
- 1 cup water
- 1/2 teaspoon ground turmeric
- 1/2 teaspoon ground ginger
- 1 tablespoon maple syrup
- 1/4 cup chopped nuts (such as almonds or walnuts)

- Fresh berries, for topping

 Instructions:
1. In a small saucepan, bring the water to a boil. Stir in the oats, turmeric, ginger, and maple syrup. Reduce heat to low and cook, stirring occasionally, for 5-7 minutes, or until the oats are tender and creamy.
2. Stir in the chopped nuts.
3. Serve the oatmeal in bowls, topped with fresh berries.

7. SWEET POTATO BREAKFAST BOWL

 Ingredients:
- 1 small sweet potato
- 1/2 tablespoon coconut oil
- 1/2 teaspoon ground cinnamon
- 1/4 cup almond milk (or your choice of plant-based milk)
- 1 tablespoon almond butter
- 1 tablespoon maple syrup
- 1/4 cup chopped nuts (such as pecans or walnuts)

 Instructions:
1. Preheat the oven to 400°F (200°C).
2. Pierce the sweet potato with a fork several times and place it on a baking sheet.
3. Bake for 45-60 minutes, or until the sweet potato is tender.
4. Remove the sweet potato from the oven and let it cool slightly.
5. Peel the skin off the sweet potato and place the flesh in a bowl.
6. Add the coconut oil, cinnamon, almond milk, almond butter, and maple syrup to the bowl. Mash everything together until well combined.
7. Serve the sweet potato mixture in a bowl, topped with chopped nuts.

8. COCONUT CHIA PUDDING

 Ingredients:
- 1/4 cup chia seeds

- 1 cup coconut milk
- 1 tablespoon maple syrup
- 1/2 teaspoon vanilla extract
- Fresh fruit, for topping
- Unsweetened shredded coconut, for garnish

Instructions:
1. In a bowl, combine the chia seeds, coconut milk, maple syrup, and vanilla extract. Stir well to combine.
2. Cover and refrigerate for at least 2 hours, or overnight, until the mixture thickens and becomes pudding-like.
3. Serve the chia pudding in bowls, topped with fresh fruit and a sprinkle of unsweetened shredded coconut.

9. BANANA ALMOND BUTTER TOAST

Ingredients:
- 2 slices whole grain bread
- 2 tablespoons almond butter
- 1 banana, sliced
- Cinnamon, for sprinkling

Instructions:
1. Toast the bread to your desired level of crispiness.
2. Spread the almond butter evenly onto each slice of toast.
3. Top the almond butter with sliced banana.
4. Sprinkle cinnamon over the banana slices.
5. Serve immediately.

10. GREEN SMOOTHIE

Ingredients:
- 1 cup spinach
- 1/2 cup kale

- 1/2 banana
- 1/2 cup frozen mixed berries
- 1 tablespoon almond butter
- 1 cup almond milk (or your choice of plant-based milk)
- 1 tablespoon chia seeds (optional)

Instructions:
1. Combine all ingredients in a blender.
2. Blend until smooth.
3. Pour into a glass and enjoy!

11. APPLE CINNAMON OATMEAL

Ingredients:
- 1/2 cup rolled oats
- 1 cup water
- 1/2 apple, chopped
- 1/2 teaspoon ground cinnamon
- 1 tablespoon maple syrup
- 1/4 cup chopped nuts (such as almonds or walnuts)

Instructions:
1. In a small saucepan, bring the water to a boil. Stir in the oats, apple, cinnamon, and maple syrup.
2. Reduce heat to low and cook, stirring occasionally, for 5-7 minutes, or until the oats are tender and creamy.
3. Stir in the chopped nuts.
4. Serve the oatmeal in bowls.

12. MANGO COCONUT CHIA PUDDING

Ingredients:
- 1/4 cup chia seeds
- 1 cup coconut milk
- 1 tablespoon maple syrup

- 1/2 teaspoon vanilla extract
- 1/2 cup chopped mango
- Unsweetened shredded coconut, for garnish

Instructions:
1. In a bowl, combine the chia seeds, coconut milk, maple syrup, and vanilla extract. Stir well to combine.
2. Cover and refrigerate for at least 2 hours, or overnight, until the mixture thickens and becomes pudding-like.
3. Serve the chia pudding in bowls, topped with chopped mango and a sprinkle of unsweetened shredded coconut.

13. PEANUT BUTTER BANANA SMOOTHIE

Ingredients:
- 1 banana
- 2 tablespoons peanut butter
- 1 cup almond milk (or your choice of plant-based milk)
- 1 tablespoon chia seeds (optional)
- 1 teaspoon honey or maple syrup (optional)

Instructions:
1. Combine all ingredients in a blender.
2. Blend until smooth.
3. Pour into a glass and enjoy!

14. CHOCOLATE AVOCADO SMOOTHIE BOWL

Ingredients:
- 1 ripe avocado
- 1 banana
- 2 tablespoons cocoa powder
- 1 cup almond milk (or your choice of plant-based milk)
- 1 tablespoon maple syrup or honey

- Toppings: sliced banana, granola, cacao nibs

Instructions:
1. Combine the avocado, banana, cocoa powder, almond milk, and maple syrup in a blender.
2. Blend until smooth.
3. Pour the smoothie into a bowl and top with sliced banana, granola, and cacao nibs.

15. ALMOND JOY OVERNIGHT OATS

Ingredients:
- 1/2 cup rolled oats
- 1/2 cup almond milk (or your choice of plant-based milk)
- 1 tablespoon cocoa powder
- 1 tablespoon maple syrup
- 1 tablespoon shredded coconut
- 1 tablespoon sliced almonds
- 1 tablespoon dairy-free chocolate chips (optional)

Instructions:
1. In a jar or container, combine the oats, almond milk, cocoa powder, and maple syrup. Stir well to combine.
2. Add the shredded coconut, sliced almonds, and chocolate chips (if using).
3. Cover and refrigerate overnight.
4. In the morning, stir the oats and add more almond milk if desired.
5. Enjoy cold or heat in the microwave before serving.

16. TURMERIC GINGER SMOOTHIE

Ingredients:
- 1 banana
- 1/2 cup pineapple chunks
- 1/2 teaspoon ground turmeric

- 1/2 teaspoon grated ginger
- 1 tablespoon chia seeds
- 1 cup coconut water or almond milk

Instructions:
1. Combine all ingredients in a blender.
2. Blend until smooth.
3. Pour into a glass and enjoy!

17. SPINACH AND MUSHROOM TOFU SCRAMBLE

Ingredients:
- 1/2 block firm tofu, crumbled
- 1 cup spinach
- 1/2 cup sliced mushrooms
- 1/4 teaspoon turmeric
- 1/4 teaspoon garlic powder
- Salt and pepper, to taste
- 1 tablespoon nutritional yeast (optional)

Instructions:
1. In a skillet over medium heat, sauté the mushrooms until they begin to soften.
2. Add the spinach and cook until wilted.
3. Add the crumbled tofu, turmeric, garlic powder, salt, and pepper. Cook for 2-3 minutes, stirring occasionally.
4. Sprinkle with nutritional yeast, if using, and serve hot.

18. BERRY CHIA SEED PUDDING PARFAIT

Ingredients:
- 1/4 cup chia seeds
- 1 cup almond milk (or your choice of plant-based milk)
- 1 tablespoon maple syrup
- 1/2 teaspoon vanilla extract

- 1/2 cup mixed berries
- Granola, for topping

Instructions:
1. In a bowl, combine the chia seeds, almond milk, maple syrup, and vanilla extract. Stir well to combine.
2. Cover and refrigerate for at least 2 hours, or overnight, until the mixture thickens and becomes pudding-like.
3. In a glass, layer the chia seed pudding with mixed berries and granola.
4. Repeat the layers until the glass is full.
5. Serve chilled.

19. SAVORY SWEET POTATO HASH

Ingredients:
- 1 large sweet potato, peeled and diced
- 1 bell pepper, diced
- 1 onion, diced
- 2 cloves garlic, minced
- 1 teaspoon smoked paprika
- 1/2 teaspoon cumin
- Salt and pepper, to taste
- 2 tablespoons olive oil
- Fresh cilantro, for garnish

Instructions:
1. Heat olive oil in a large skillet over medium heat.
2. Add sweet potato and cook for about 5 minutes, stirring occasionally.
3. Add bell pepper, onion, and garlic. Cook for another 5-7 minutes, or until vegetables are tender.
4. Add smoked paprika, cumin, salt, and pepper. Stir to combine.
5. Cook for an additional 2-3 minutes.
6. Garnish with fresh cilantro before serving.

20. COCONUT CHIA SEED PUDDING WITH MANGO

Ingredients:
- 1/4 cup chia seeds
- 1 cup coconut milk
- 1 tablespoon maple syrup
- 1/2 teaspoon vanilla extract
- 1 ripe mango, diced
- Unsweetened shredded coconut, for garnish

Instructions:
1. In a bowl, combine chia seeds, coconut milk, maple syrup, and vanilla extract. Stir well.
2. Cover and refrigerate for at least 2 hours or overnight, until the mixture thickens.
3. In a serving glass, layer chia seed pudding with diced mango.
4. Repeat the layers until the glass is full.
5. Sprinkle with shredded coconut before serving.

21. AVOCADO AND BLACK BEAN WRAP

Ingredients:
- 1 whole grain wrap
- 1/2 avocado, mashed
- 1/4 cup black beans, drained and rinsed
- 2 tablespoons salsa
- Handful of spinach leaves
- Salt and pepper, to taste

Instructions:
1. Lay the wrap flat on a plate.
2. Spread mashed avocado evenly over the wrap.
3. Top with black beans, salsa, spinach leaves, salt, and pepper.
4. Roll up the wrap tightly.
5. Slice in half and serve.

Chapter 2: Lunch Recipes

22. MEDITERRANEAN QUINOA SALAD

Ingredients:
- 1 cup quinoa, cooked
- 1/2 cucumber, diced
- 1/2 red bell pepper, diced
- 1/4 cup red onion, finely chopped
- 1/4 cup Kalamata olives, sliced
- 1/4 cup fresh parsley, chopped
- 1/4 cup crumbled feta cheese (optional)
- 2 tablespoons olive oil
- 1 tablespoon lemon juice
- 1 teaspoon dried oregano
- Salt and pepper, to taste

Instructions:
1. In a large bowl, combine quinoa, cucumber, bell pepper, onion, olives, and parsley.
2. In a small bowl, whisk together olive oil, lemon juice, oregano, salt, and pepper.
3. Pour the dressing over the quinoa salad and toss to combine.
4. Sprinkle with feta cheese, if using, before serving.

23. VEGGIE STIR-FRY WITH TOFU

Ingredients:
- 1 block firm tofu, drained and cubed
- 2 tablespoons soy sauce
- 1 tablespoon sesame oil
- 1 tablespoon olive oil
- 2 cloves garlic, minced
- 1 tablespoon ginger, minced
- 1 bell pepper, sliced

- 1 zucchini, sliced
- 1 carrot, julienned
- 1 cup broccoli florets
- Cooked brown rice, for serving

Instructions:
1. In a bowl, marinate tofu cubes in soy sauce for 15-20 minutes.
2. Heat olive oil in a large skillet over medium heat.
3. Add garlic and ginger, and sauté for 1-2 minutes.
4. Add marinated tofu to the skillet and cook until browned on all sides.
5. Add bell pepper, zucchini, carrot, and broccoli to the skillet. Cook until vegetables are tender-crisp.
6. Serve the stir-fry over cooked brown rice.

24. LENTIL AND VEGETABLE SOUP

Ingredients:
- 1 cup dried lentils, rinsed and drained
- 4 cups vegetable broth
- 1 onion, chopped
- 2 carrots, chopped
- 2 celery stalks, chopped
- 2 cloves garlic, minced
- 1 teaspoon dried thyme
- 1 teaspoon dried rosemary
- Salt and pepper, to taste
- Fresh parsley, for garnish

Instructions:
1. In a large pot, combine lentils, vegetable broth, onion, carrots, celery, garlic, thyme, and rosemary.
2. Bring to a boil, then reduce heat and simmer for 25-30 minutes, or until lentils are tender.
3. Season with salt and pepper.
4. Serve hot, garnished with fresh parsley.

25. CHICKPEA AVOCADO SALAD WRAP

Ingredients:
- 1 can (15 oz) chickpeas, drained and rinsed
- 1 avocado, mashed
- 1/4 cup red onion, finely chopped
- 1/4 cup bell pepper, diced
- 1/4 cup cucumber, diced
- 1 tablespoon lemon juice
- 1 tablespoon olive oil
- Salt and pepper, to taste
- Whole grain wraps

Instructions:
1. In a large bowl, combine chickpeas, mashed avocado, red onion, bell pepper, cucumber, lemon juice, olive oil, salt, and pepper. Mix well.
2. Place a generous scoop of the chickpea avocado salad onto a whole grain wrap.
3. Roll up the wrap tightly and cut in half.
4. Serve immediately or wrap in foil for later.

26. MEXICAN QUINOA STUFFED BELL PEPPERS

Ingredients:
- 4 bell peppers, halved and seeds removed
- 1 cup quinoa, cooked
- 1 can (15 oz) black beans, drained and rinsed
- 1 cup corn kernels
- 1/2 cup salsa
- 1 teaspoon chili powder
- 1/2 teaspoon cumin
- Salt and pepper, to taste
- 1/2 cup shredded vegan cheese (optional)
- Fresh cilantro, for garnish

Instructions:
1. Preheat the oven to 375°F (190°C).
2. In a large bowl, combine cooked quinoa, black beans, corn, salsa, chili powder, cumin, salt, and pepper.
3. Spoon the quinoa mixture into each bell pepper half.
4. Place the stuffed bell peppers in a baking dish.
5. Cover the dish with foil and bake for 25-30 minutes, or until the bell peppers are tender.
6. Remove the foil, sprinkle vegan cheese on top of each bell pepper, and bake for an additional 5 minutes, or until the cheese is melted.
7. Garnish with fresh cilantro before serving.

27. CURRIED CHICKPEA SALAD SANDWICH

Ingredients:
- 1 can (15 oz) chickpeas, drained and rinsed
- 1/4 cup vegan mayonnaise
- 1 tablespoon curry powder
- 1/4 cup celery, finely chopped
- 1/4 cup red onion, finely chopped
- Salt and pepper, to taste
- Whole grain bread
- Lettuce leaves, for serving
- Sliced tomatoes, for serving

Instructions:
1. In a bowl, mash the chickpeas with a fork or potato masher.
2. Add vegan mayonnaise, curry powder, celery, red onion, salt, and pepper. Mix well.
3. Spread the chickpea salad onto whole grain bread slices.
4. Top with lettuce leaves and sliced tomatoes.
5. Close the sandwich and serve.

28. SWEET POTATO AND BLACK BEAN QUESADILLAS

Ingredients:
- 2 large sweet potatoes, peeled and diced
- 1 can (15 oz) black beans, drained and rinsed
- 1 teaspoon ground cumin
- 1 teaspoon smoked paprika
- Salt and pepper, to taste
- 4 whole grain tortillas
- 1 cup shredded vegan cheese
- Salsa, guacamole, and vegan sour cream, for serving

Instructions:
1. Preheat the oven to 400°F (200°C).
2. Place the diced sweet potatoes on a baking sheet. Drizzle with olive oil, cumin, smoked paprika, salt, and pepper. Toss to coat.
3. Roast the sweet potatoes for 20-25 minutes, or until tender.
4. In a bowl, mash half of the black beans with a fork. Leave the other half whole.
5. Lay out the tortillas and divide the mashed black beans, whole black beans, roasted sweet potatoes, and vegan cheese evenly among them.
6. Fold the tortillas in half to form quesadillas.
7. Heat a large skillet over medium heat. Cook the quesadillas for 3-4 minutes per side, or until golden brown and crispy.
8. Serve the quesadillas with salsa, guacamole, and vegan sour cream.

29. RAINBOW SPRING ROLLS WITH PEANUT DIPPING SAUCE

Ingredients:
- 8 rice paper wrappers
- 1 large carrot, julienned
- 1 cucumber, julienned
- 1 bell pepper, thinly sliced
- 1/2 cup purple cabbage, thinly sliced
- 1/2 cup fresh cilantro leaves

- 1/2 cup fresh mint leaves
- 1/2 cup cooked rice noodles (optional)
- Peanut dipping sauce (see recipe below)

Instructions:
1. Fill a shallow dish with warm water. Dip one rice paper wrapper into the water and let it soften for about 10-15 seconds.
2. Place the softened rice paper wrapper on a clean surface.
3. Arrange a small handful of each vegetable, cilantro, mint, and rice noodles (if using) in the center of the wrapper.
4. Fold the sides of the wrapper over the filling, then roll up tightly from the bottom.
5. Repeat with the remaining wrappers and filling ingredients.
6. Serve the spring rolls with peanut dipping sauce.

30. GARDEN VEGETABLE SOUP

Ingredients:
- 1 tablespoon olive oil
- 1 onion, chopped
- 2 carrots, diced
- 2 celery stalks, diced
- 2 cloves garlic, minced
- 1 zucchini, diced
- 1 yellow squash, diced
- 1 can (15 oz) diced tomatoes
- 4 cups vegetable broth
- 1 teaspoon dried thyme
- 1 teaspoon dried basil
- Salt and pepper, to taste
- Fresh parsley, for garnish

Instructions:
1. Heat olive oil in a large pot over medium heat.

2. Add onion, carrots, and celery. Cook until vegetables are softened, about 5-7 minutes.
3. Add garlic, zucchini, and yellow squash. Cook for another 2-3 minutes.
4. Stir in diced tomatoes, vegetable broth, thyme, basil, salt, and pepper.
5. Bring to a simmer and cook for 15-20 minutes, or until vegetables are tender.
6. Serve hot, garnished with fresh parsley.

31. CHICKPEA AVOCADO SALAD

Ingredients:
- 1 can (15 oz) chickpeas, drained and rinsed
- 1 avocado, diced
- 1/4 cup red onion, finely chopped
- 1/4 cup cucumber, diced
- 1/4 cup bell pepper, diced
- 2 tablespoons fresh cilantro, chopped
- Juice of 1 lime
- Salt and pepper, to taste

Instructions:
1. In a large bowl, combine chickpeas, avocado, red onion, cucumber, bell pepper, and cilantro.
2. Add lime juice, salt, and pepper. Mix well to combine.
3. Serve as a salad or in a wrap.

32. MEXICAN QUINOA SALAD

Ingredients:
- 1 cup quinoa, cooked
- 1 can (15 oz) black beans, drained and rinsed
- 1 cup corn kernels
- 1/2 cup cherry tomatoes, halved
- 1/4 cup red onion, finely chopped

- 1/4 cup fresh cilantro, chopped
- Juice of 1 lime
- 1 teaspoon cumin
- Salt and pepper, to taste
- Avocado, for serving (optional)

Instructions:
1. In a large bowl, combine quinoa, black beans, corn, cherry tomatoes, red onion, and cilantro.
2. Add lime juice, cumin, salt, and pepper. Mix well to combine.
3. Serve topped with sliced avocado, if desired.

33. LENTIL AND VEGETABLE STIR-FRY

Ingredients:
- 1 cup lentils, cooked
- 1 tablespoon sesame oil
- 2 cloves garlic, minced
- 1 tablespoon ginger, minced
- 1 bell pepper, sliced
- 1 zucchini, sliced
- 1 carrot, julienned
- 1/4 cup soy sauce
- 2 tablespoons rice vinegar
- 1 tablespoon maple syrup
- Cooked brown rice, for serving

Instructions:
1. Heat sesame oil in a large skillet over medium heat.
2. Add garlic and ginger, and sauté for 1-2 minutes.
3. Add bell pepper, zucchini, and carrot. Cook until vegetables are tender-crisp.
4. Stir in lentils, soy sauce, rice vinegar, and maple syrup. Cook for another 2-3 minutes.
5. Serve over cooked brown rice.

34. CAPRESE STUFFED AVOCADOS

Ingredients:
- 2 avocados, halved and pitted
- 1 cup cherry tomatoes, halved
- 1/2 cup fresh basil leaves, chopped
- 1/2 cup fresh mozzarella, diced
- Balsamic glaze, for drizzling
- Salt and pepper, to taste

Instructions:
1. Scoop out some flesh from each avocado half to create a larger cavity.
2. In a bowl, combine cherry tomatoes, basil, and mozzarella. Season with salt and pepper.
3. Stuff each avocado half with the tomato mixture.
4. Drizzle with balsamic glaze before serving.

35. VEGGIE AND HUMMUS WRAP

Ingredients:
- 1 whole grain wrap
- 2 tablespoons hummus
- 1/4 cup shredded carrots
- 1/4 cup cucumber, sliced
- 1/4 cup bell pepper, sliced
- Handful of spinach leaves

Instructions:
1. Spread hummus evenly onto the whole grain wrap.
2. Layer shredded carrots, cucumber, bell pepper, and spinach leaves on top of the hummus.
3. Roll up the wrap tightly and cut in half.
4. Serve immediately or wrap in foil for later.

36. PUMPKIN CHILI

Ingredients:
- 1 tablespoon olive oil
- 1 onion, chopped
- 2 cloves garlic, minced
- 1 bell pepper, chopped
- 1 can (15 oz) pumpkin puree
- 1 can (15 oz) black beans, drained and rinsed
- 1 can (15 oz) diced tomatoes
- 2 cups vegetable broth
- 1 tablespoon chili powder
- 1 teaspoon cumin
- Salt and pepper, to taste
- Fresh cilantro, for garnish

Instructions:
1. Heat olive oil in a large pot over medium heat.
2. Add onion, garlic, and bell pepper. Cook until vegetables are softened, about 5-7 minutes.
3. Stir in pumpkin puree, black beans, diced tomatoes, vegetable broth, chili powder, cumin, salt, and pepper.
4. Bring to a simmer and cook for 15-20 minutes, stirring occasionally.
5. Serve hot, garnished with fresh cilantro.

37. MEDITERRANEAN BUDDHA BOWL

Ingredients:
- 1 cup cooked quinoa
- 1/2 cup chickpeas, drained and rinsed
- 1/2 cucumber, diced
- 1/2 cup cherry tomatoes, halved
- 1/4 cup red onion, finely chopped
- 1/4 cup Kalamata olives, sliced
- 1/4 cup crumbled feta cheese (optional)

- 2 tablespoons hummus
- Fresh parsley, for garnish
- Lemon wedges, for serving

Instructions:
1. In a bowl, layer cooked quinoa, chickpeas, cucumber, cherry tomatoes, red onion, and Kalamata olives.
2. Top with crumbled feta cheese, if using, and a dollop of hummus.
3. Garnish with fresh parsley and serve with lemon wedges.

38. SWEET POTATO BLACK BEAN QUESADILLA

Ingredients:
- 2 large sweet potatoes, peeled and diced
- 1 can (15 oz) black beans, drained and rinsed
- 1 teaspoon ground cumin
- 1 teaspoon smoked paprika
- Salt and pepper, to taste
- 4 whole grain tortillas
- 1 cup shredded vegan cheese
- Salsa, guacamole, and vegan sour cream, for serving

Instructions:
1. Preheat the oven to 400°F (200°C).
2. Place the diced sweet potatoes on a baking sheet. Drizzle with olive oil, cumin, smoked paprika, salt, and pepper. Toss to coat.
3. Roast the sweet potatoes for 20-25 minutes, or until tender.
4. In a bowl, mash half of the black beans with a fork. Leave the other half whole.
5. Lay out the tortillas and divide the mashed black beans, whole black beans, roasted sweet potatoes, and vegan cheese evenly among them.
6. Fold the tortillas in half to form quesadillas.
7. Heat a large skillet over medium heat. Cook the quesadillas for 3-4 minutes per side, or until golden brown and crispy.
8. Serve the quesadillas with salsa, guacamole, and vegan sour cream.

39. RAINBOW SPRING ROLLS WITH PEANUT SAUCE

Ingredients:
- 8 rice paper wrappers
- 1 large carrot, julienned
- 1/2 cucumber, julienned
- 1/2 bell pepper, thinly sliced
- 1/2 cup purple cabbage, thinly sliced
- 1/2 cup fresh mint leaves
- 1/2 cup fresh cilantro leaves
- 1/2 cup cooked rice vermicelli noodles
- Peanut sauce, for serving (see recipe below)

Instructions:
1. Fill a large shallow dish with warm water. Dip one rice paper wrapper into the water and let it soften for about 10-15 seconds.
2. Place the softened rice paper wrapper on a clean surface.
3. Arrange a small handful of each vegetable, mint leaves, cilantro leaves, and rice vermicelli noodles in the center of the wrapper.
4. Fold the sides of the wrapper over the filling, then roll up tightly from the bottom.
5. Repeat with the remaining wrappers and filling ingredients.
6. Serve the spring rolls with peanut sauce.

40. GARDEN VEGETABLE SOUP

Ingredients:
- 1 tablespoon olive oil
- 1 onion, chopped
- 2 carrots, diced
- 2 celery stalks, diced
- 2 cloves garlic, minced
- 1 zucchini, diced
- 1 yellow squash, diced

- 1 can (15 oz) diced tomatoes
- 4 cups vegetable broth
- 1 teaspoon dried thyme
- 1 teaspoon dried basil
- Salt and pepper, to taste
- Fresh parsley, for garnish

Instructions:
1. Heat olive oil in a large pot over medium heat.
2. Add onion, carrots, and celery. Cook until vegetables are softened, about 5-7 minutes.
3. Add garlic, zucchini, and yellow squash. Cook for another 2-3 minutes.
4. Stir in diced tomatoes, vegetable broth, thyme, basil, salt, and pepper.
5. Bring to a simmer and cook for 15-20 minutes, or until vegetables are tender.
6. Serve hot, garnished with fresh parsley.

41. BLACK BEAN AND SWEET POTATO BURRITO BOWL

Ingredients:
- 1 cup cooked brown rice
- 1 can (15 oz) black beans, drained and rinsed
- 1 large sweet potato, peeled and diced
- 1 teaspoon ground cumin
- 1 teaspoon smoked paprika
- Salt and pepper, to taste
- 1/2 avocado, sliced
- Fresh cilantro, for garnish
- Lime wedges, for serving

Instructions:
1. In a large skillet, combine black beans, cooked brown rice, ground cumin, smoked paprika, salt, and pepper. Cook over medium heat until heated through.
2. In a separate skillet, cook the diced sweet potato until tender.

3. To assemble the burrito bowls, divide the black bean and rice mixture, cooked sweet potato, avocado slices, and fresh cilantro among bowls.
4. Serve with lime wedges.

42. VEGGIE PITA SANDWICH WITH HUMMUS

Ingredients:
- 1 whole wheat pita bread
- 2 tablespoons hummus
- 1/4 cup shredded carrots
- 1/4 cup sliced cucumber
- 1/4 cup sliced bell pepper
- Handful of spinach leaves

Instructions:
1. Cut the pita bread in half to form pockets.
2. Spread hummus inside each pocket.
3. Fill each pocket with shredded carrots, cucumber, bell pepper, and spinach leaves.
4. Serve immediately.

Chapter 3: Dinner Recipes

43. CHICKPEA COCONUT CURRY

Ingredients:
- 1 tablespoon coconut oil
- 1 onion, chopped
- 2 cloves garlic, minced
- 1 tablespoon ginger, minced
- 1 bell pepper, chopped
- 1 zucchini, chopped
- 1 carrot, sliced
- 1 can (15 oz) chickpeas, drained and rinsed
- 1 can (14 oz) coconut milk
- 2 tablespoons red curry paste
- 1 tablespoon soy sauce
- 1 tablespoon maple syrup
- Salt and pepper, to taste
- Fresh cilantro, for garnish
- Cooked rice, for serving

Instructions:
1. Heat coconut oil in a large skillet over medium heat.
2. Add onion, garlic, and ginger. Sauté for 2-3 minutes, or until fragrant.
3. Add bell pepper, zucchini, and carrot. Cook for another 5 minutes, or until vegetables begin to soften.
4. Stir in chickpeas, coconut milk, red curry paste, soy sauce, maple syrup, salt, and pepper.
5. Bring to a simmer and cook for 15-20 minutes, stirring occasionally.
6. Serve hot over cooked rice, garnished with fresh cilantro.

44. SPINACH AND MUSHROOM STUFFED SWEET POTATOES

Ingredients:
- 4 large sweet potatoes

- 2 tablespoons olive oil
- 1 onion, chopped
- 2 cloves garlic, minced
- 8 oz mushrooms, sliced
- 4 cups spinach
- 1/2 teaspoon dried thyme
- Salt and pepper, to taste
- Vegan cheese, for topping (optional)

Instructions:
1. Preheat the oven to 400°F (200°C).
2. Pierce sweet potatoes with a fork and place them on a baking sheet. Bake for 45-60 minutes, or until tender.
3. In a large skillet, heat olive oil over medium heat.
4. Add onion and garlic. Sauté for 2-3 minutes, or until softened.
5. Add mushrooms and cook for another 5 minutes, or until mushrooms are tender.
6. Add spinach, thyme, salt, and pepper. Cook until spinach is wilted.
7. Cut a slit in each sweet potato and fluff the flesh with a fork.
8. Spoon the spinach and mushroom mixture into each sweet potato.
9. Top with vegan cheese, if using.
10. Bake for an additional 5 minutes, or until the cheese is melted.
11. Serve hot.

45. LENTIL SHEPHERD'S PIE

Ingredients:
- 1 cup green lentils, rinsed and drained
- 2 cups vegetable broth
- 1 onion, chopped
- 2 carrots, diced
- 2 celery stalks, diced
- 2 cloves garlic, minced
- 1 teaspoon dried thyme
- 1 teaspoon dried rosemary

- Salt and pepper, to taste
- 4 cups mashed potatoes

 Instructions:
1. Preheat the oven to 400°F (200°C).
2. In a large pot, combine lentils and vegetable broth. Bring to a boil, then reduce heat and simmer for 20-25 minutes, or until lentils are tender.
3. In a skillet, heat olive oil over medium heat.
4. Add onion, carrots, celery, and garlic. Sauté for 5-7 minutes, or until vegetables are softened.
5. Add cooked lentils, thyme, rosemary, salt, and pepper to the skillet. Cook for another 5 minutes.
6. Spoon the lentil mixture into a baking dish.
7. Spread mashed potatoes over the lentil mixture.
8. Bake for 20-25 minutes, or until the mashed potatoes are lightly browned.
9. Serve hot.

46. QUINOA STUFFED BELL PEPPERS

 Ingredients:
- 4 bell peppers, halved and seeds removed
- 1 cup quinoa, cooked
- 1 can (15 oz) black beans, drained and rinsed
- 1 cup corn kernels
- 1/2 cup salsa
- 1 teaspoon chili powder
- 1/2 teaspoon cumin
- Salt and pepper, to taste
- Vegan cheese, for topping (optional)
- Fresh cilantro, for garnish

 Instructions:
1. Preheat the oven to 375°F (190°C).

2. In a large bowl, combine cooked quinoa, black beans, corn, salsa, chili powder, cumin, salt, and pepper.
3. Spoon the quinoa mixture into each bell pepper half.
4. Place the stuffed bell peppers in a baking dish.
5. Cover the dish with foil and bake for 25-30 minutes, or until the bell peppers are tender.
6. Remove the foil, sprinkle vegan cheese on top of each bell pepper, and bake for an additional 5 minutes, or until the cheese is melted and bubbly.
7. Remove from the oven and let cool for a few minutes.
8. Garnish with fresh cilantro before serving. Enjoy your delicious and nutritious quinoa stuffed bell peppers!

47. MOROCCAN-SPICED VEGETABLE TAGINE

Ingredients:
- 2 tablespoons olive oil
- 1 onion, chopped
- 2 cloves garlic, minced
- 1 tablespoon fresh ginger, minced
- 1 teaspoon ground cumin
- 1 teaspoon ground coriander
- 1/2 teaspoon ground cinnamon
- 1/2 teaspoon ground turmeric
- 1/4 teaspoon cayenne pepper
- 1 can (15 oz) chickpeas, drained and rinsed
- 1 can (14 oz) diced tomatoes
- 2 cups vegetable broth
- 1 sweet potato, peeled and diced
- 2 carrots, peeled and sliced
- 1 zucchini, diced
- 1/2 cup dried apricots, chopped
- Salt and pepper, to taste
- Cooked couscous, for serving
- Fresh cilantro, for garnish

Instructions:
1. Heat olive oil in a large pot over medium heat.
2. Add onion and cook until softened, about 5 minutes.
3. Stir in garlic, ginger, cumin, coriander, cinnamon, turmeric, and cayenne pepper. Cook for another 2 minutes, or until fragrant.
4. Add chickpeas, diced tomatoes, vegetable broth, sweet potato, carrots, zucchini, and dried apricots to the pot.
5. Season with salt and pepper. Bring to a simmer.
6. Cover and cook for 20-25 minutes, or until vegetables are tender.
7. Serve over cooked couscous, garnished with fresh cilantro.

48. VEGETABLE PAD THAI

Ingredients:
- 8 oz rice noodles
- 2 tablespoons soy sauce
- 2 tablespoons tamarind paste
- 2 tablespoons maple syrup
- 1 tablespoon rice vinegar
- 1 tablespoon sriracha sauce
- 2 tablespoons vegetable oil
- 1 onion, thinly sliced
- 2 cloves garlic, minced
- 1 bell pepper, thinly sliced
- 1 cup broccoli florets
- 1 carrot, julienned
- 1/2 cup bean sprouts
- 1/4 cup chopped peanuts
- Lime wedges, for serving
- Fresh cilantro, for garnish

Instructions:
1. Cook rice noodles according to package instructions. Drain and set aside.
2. In a small bowl, whisk together soy sauce, tamarind paste, maple syrup, rice vinegar, and sriracha sauce. Set aside.

3. Heat vegetable oil in a large skillet over medium heat.

4. Add onion and garlic. Cook until softened, about 5 minutes.

5. Add bell pepper, broccoli, and carrot. Cook for another 5 minutes, or until vegetables are tender-crisp.

6. Stir in cooked rice noodles and sauce mixture. Cook for 2-3 minutes, or until heated through.

7. Serve hot, garnished with bean sprouts, chopped peanuts, lime wedges, and fresh cilantro.

49. MUSHROOM STROGANOFF

Ingredients:
- 8 oz pasta of choice
- 2 tablespoons olive oil
- 1 onion, chopped
- 2 cloves garlic, minced
- 8 oz mushrooms, sliced
- 2 tablespoons flour
- 1 cup vegetable broth
- 1 tablespoon soy sauce
- 1/2 cup vegan sour cream
- Salt and pepper, to taste
- Fresh parsley, for garnish

Instructions:
1. Cook pasta according to package instructions. Drain and set aside.

2. In a large skillet, heat olive oil over medium heat.

3. Add onion and garlic. Cook until softened, about 5 minutes.

4. Add mushrooms and cook for another 5 minutes, or until mushrooms are tender.

5. Sprinkle flour over the mushroom mixture and stir to combine.

6. Gradually whisk in vegetable broth and soy sauce. Cook until thickened, about 5 minutes.

7. Remove from heat and stir in vegan sour cream. Season with salt and pepper.

8. Serve over cooked pasta, garnished with fresh parsley.

50. STUFFED ACORN SQUASH

Ingredients:
- 2 acorn squash, halved and seeds removed
- 2 tablespoons olive oil
- 1 onion, chopped
- 2 cloves garlic, minced
- 1 bell pepper, chopped
- 1 zucchini, chopped
- 1 cup cooked quinoa
- 1 can (15 oz) black beans, drained and rinsed
- 1 teaspoon ground cumin
- 1 teaspoon smoked paprika
- Salt and pepper, to taste
- Vegan cheese, for topping (optional)
- Fresh cilantro, for garnish

Instructions:
1. Preheat the oven to 400°F (200°C).
2. Place acorn squash halves cut-side down on a baking sheet. Bake for 30-35 minutes, or until tender.
3. In a large skillet, heat olive oil over medium heat.
4. Add onion and garlic. Cook until softened, about 5 minutes.
5. Add bell pepper and zucchini. Cook for another 5 minutes, or until vegetables are tender.
6. Stir in cooked quinoa, black beans, cumin, smoked paprika, salt, and pepper.
7. Divide the quinoa mixture among the acorn squash halves.
8. Top with vegan cheese, if using.
9. Bake for an additional 10 minutes, or until heated through.
10. Serve hot, garnished with fresh cilantro.

51. VEGAN JAMBALAYA

Ingredients:
- 1 tablespoon olive oil
- 1 onion, chopped
- 2 cloves garlic, minced
- 1 bell pepper, chopped
- 2 celery stalks, chopped
- 1 can (14 oz) diced tomatoes
- 1 cup vegetable broth
- 1 teaspoon smoked paprika
- 1 teaspoon dried thyme
- 1/2 teaspoon cayenne pepper
- 1 cup long-grain white rice
- 1 can (15 oz) kidney beans, drained and rinsed
- 1 cup sliced okra
- Salt and pepper, to taste
- Fresh parsley, for garnish

Instructions:
1. Heat olive oil in a large pot over medium heat.
2. Add onion, garlic, bell pepper, and celery. Cook until softened, about 5 minutes.
3. Stir in diced tomatoes, vegetable broth, smoked paprika, thyme, and cayenne pepper.
4. Bring to a simmer and add rice. Cover and cook for 15-20 minutes, or until rice is almost tender.
5. Stir in kidney beans and okra. Cook for another 5-10 minutes, or until rice and vegetables are tender.
6. Season with salt and pepper. Serve hot, garnished with fresh parsley.

52. VEGETABLE AND WHITE BEAN STEW

Ingredients:
- 1 tablespoon olive oil
- 1 onion, chopped
- 2 cloves garlic, minced
- 2 carrots, chopped
- 2 celery stalks, chopped
- 1 bell pepper, chopped
- 1 can (14 oz) diced tomatoes
- 4 cups vegetable broth
- 1 can (15 oz) white beans, drained and rinsed
- 1 teaspoon dried thyme
- 1 teaspoon dried rosemary
- Salt and pepper, to taste
- Fresh parsley, for garnish

Instructions:
1. Heat olive oil in a large pot over medium heat.
2. Add onion and garlic. Cook until softened, about 5 minutes.
3. Stir in carrots, celery, and bell pepper. Cook for another 5 minutes.
4. Add diced tomatoes, vegetable broth, white beans, thyme, and rosemary.
5. Bring to a simmer and cook for 20-25 minutes, or until vegetables are tender.
6. Season with salt and pepper. Serve hot, garnished with fresh parsley.

53. VEGAN MOUSSAKA

Ingredients:
- 2 eggplants, sliced
- 2 tablespoons olive oil
- 1 onion, chopped
- 2 cloves garlic, minced
- 1 can (14 oz) diced tomatoes
- 1 can (15 oz) lentils, drained and rinsed
- 1 teaspoon dried oregano
- 1 teaspoon ground cinnamon

- Salt and pepper, to taste
- 2 cups vegan bechamel sauce
- Vegan cheese, for topping (optional)
- Fresh parsley, for garnish

Instructions:
1. Preheat the oven to 400°F (200°C).
2. Place eggplant slices on a baking sheet. Drizzle with olive oil and season with salt and pepper. Roast in the oven for 20-25 minutes, or until tender.
3. In a large skillet, heat olive oil over medium heat.
4. Add onion and garlic. Cook until softened, about 5 minutes.
5. Stir in diced tomatoes, lentils, oregano, cinnamon, salt, and pepper.
6. Simmer for 10-15 minutes, or until thickened.
7. In a baking dish, layer roasted eggplant slices and lentil mixture. Repeat layers.
8. Pour vegan bechamel sauce over the top and spread evenly.
9. Sprinkle vegan cheese on top, if using.
10. Bake for 30-35 minutes, or until bubbly and golden.
11. Serve hot, garnished with fresh parsley.

54. THAI PEANUT SWEET POTATO BUDDHA BOWL

Ingredients:
- 2 sweet potatoes, peeled and cubed
- 1 tablespoon olive oil
- 1 can (15 oz) chickpeas, drained and rinsed
- 1/4 cup peanut butter
- 2 tablespoons soy sauce
- 1 tablespoon maple syrup
- 1 tablespoon rice vinegar
- 1 teaspoon sriracha sauce
- Cooked quinoa, for serving
- Fresh cilantro, for garnish

Instructions:

1. Preheat the oven to 400°F (200°C).

2. Place sweet potato cubes on a baking sheet. Drizzle with olive oil and season with salt and pepper. Roast in the oven for 25-30 minutes, or until tender.

3. In a skillet, heat olive oil over medium heat. Add chickpeas and cook until slightly crispy, about 5-7 minutes.

4. In a small bowl, whisk together peanut butter, soy sauce, maple syrup, rice vinegar, and sriracha sauce.

5. To assemble the bowls, divide cooked quinoa among bowls. Top with roasted sweet potatoes, crispy chickpeas, and peanut sauce.

6. Serve hot, garnished with fresh cilantro.

55. VEGETABLE PAELLA

Ingredients:
- 2 tablespoons olive oil
- 1 onion, chopped
- 2 cloves garlic, minced
- 1 bell pepper, chopped
- 1 zucchini, chopped
- 1 cup diced tomatoes
- 1 teaspoon smoked paprika
- 1 teaspoon turmeric
- 1/2 teaspoon saffron threads
- 1 1/2 cups Arborio rice
- 4 cups vegetable broth
- 1 can (15 oz) artichoke hearts, drained and quartered
- 1 cup frozen peas
- Salt and pepper, to taste
- Lemon wedges, for serving
- Fresh parsley, for garnish

Instructions:
1. Heat olive oil in a large skillet or paella pan over medium heat.
2. Add onion and garlic. Cook until softened, about 5 minutes.

3. Stir in bell pepper and zucchini. Cook for another 5 minutes.
4. Add diced tomatoes, smoked paprika, turmeric, and saffron threads. Cook for 2-3 minutes.
5. Stir in Arborio rice and cook for another 2 minutes.
6. Pour in vegetable broth and bring to a simmer. Cook for 20-25 minutes, or until rice is tender and liquid is absorbed.
7. Stir in artichoke hearts and frozen peas. Cook for another 5 minutes, or until heated through.
8. Season with salt and pepper. Serve hot, with lemon wedges and fresh parsley.

56. VEGAN SWEET POTATO AND BLACK BEAN ENCHILADAS

Ingredients:
- 2 large sweet potatoes, peeled and diced
- 1 tablespoon olive oil
- 1 onion, chopped
- 2 cloves garlic, minced
- 1 bell pepper, chopped
- 1 can (15 oz) black beans, drained and rinsed
- 1 teaspoon ground cumin
- 1 teaspoon chili powder
- Salt and pepper, to taste
- 8-10 small corn tortillas
- 1 can (15 oz) enchilada sauce
- Vegan cheese, for topping (optional)
- Fresh cilantro, for garnish

Instructions:
1. Preheat the oven to 375°F (190°C).
2. Place diced sweet potatoes on a baking sheet. Drizzle with olive oil and season with salt and pepper. Roast in the oven for 20-25 minutes, or until tender.

3. In a large skillet, heat olive oil over medium heat. Add onion and garlic. Cook until softened, about 5 minutes.

4. Stir in bell pepper, black beans, cumin, chili powder, salt, and pepper. Cook for another 5 minutes.

5. To assemble the enchiladas, spread a thin layer of enchilada sauce on the bottom of a baking dish.

6. Fill each tortilla with a spoonful of the sweet potato mixture. Roll up and place seam-side down in the baking dish.

7. Pour the remaining enchilada sauce over the top of the enchiladas. Sprinkle with vegan cheese, if using.

8. Bake for 20-25 minutes, or until heated through and the cheese is melted.

9. Serve hot, garnished with fresh cilantro.

57. LEMON GARLIC ORZO WITH ROASTED VEGETABLES

Ingredients:
- 1 cup orzo pasta
- 1 tablespoon olive oil
- 1 onion, chopped
- 2 cloves garlic, minced
- 1 zucchini, chopped
- 1 yellow squash, chopped
- 1 red bell pepper, chopped
- 1 yellow bell pepper, chopped
- 1/2 cup cherry tomatoes, halved
- 1 lemon, juiced and zested
- 2 tablespoons chopped fresh parsley
- Salt and pepper, to taste

Instructions:
1. Cook orzo pasta according to package instructions. Drain and set aside.
2. Preheat the oven to 400°F (200°C).
3. Place chopped zucchini, yellow squash, red bell pepper, yellow bell pepper, and cherry tomatoes on a baking sheet. Drizzle with olive oil and

season with salt and pepper. Roast in the oven for 20-25 minutes, or until vegetables are tender.

4. In a large skillet, heat olive oil over medium heat. Add onion and garlic. Cook until softened, about 5 minutes.

5. Stir in cooked orzo, roasted vegetables, lemon juice, lemon zest, and parsley. Cook for another 2-3 minutes, or until heated through.

6. Season with salt and pepper. Serve hot.

58. VEGAN MEXICAN QUINOA STUFFED PEPPERS

Ingredients:
- 4 bell peppers, halved and seeds removed
- 1 cup quinoa, cooked
- 1 can (15 oz) black beans, drained and rinsed
- 1 cup corn kernels
- 1 can (14 oz) diced tomatoes
- 1 teaspoon ground cumin
- 1 teaspoon chili powder
- Salt and pepper, to taste
- Fresh cilantro, for garnish
- Lime wedges, for serving

Instructions:
1. Preheat the oven to 375°F (190°C).
2. Place bell pepper halves in a baking dish.
3. In a large bowl, combine cooked quinoa, black beans, corn kernels, diced tomatoes, cumin, chili powder, salt, and pepper.
4. Spoon the quinoa mixture into each bell pepper half.
5. Cover the baking dish with foil and bake for 25-30 minutes, or until bell peppers are tender.
6. Serve hot, garnished with fresh cilantro and lime wedges.

59. VEGAN CREAMY TOMATO BASIL PASTA

Ingredients:

- 8 oz pasta of choice
- 1 tablespoon olive oil
- 1 onion, chopped
- 2 cloves garlic, minced
- 1 can (14 oz) diced tomatoes
- 1/2 cup raw cashews, soaked
- 1/2 cup vegetable broth
- 1/4 cup nutritional yeast
- 1 teaspoon dried basil
- Salt and pepper, to taste
- Fresh basil, for garnish

Instructions:
1. Cook pasta according to package instructions. Drain and set aside.
2. In a large skillet, heat olive oil over medium heat. Add onion and garlic. Cook until softened, about 5 minutes.
3. Stir in diced tomatoes and cook for another 5 minutes.
4. In a blender, combine soaked cashews, vegetable broth, nutritional yeast, dried basil, salt, and pepper. Blend until smooth.
5. Pour the cashew sauce over the tomato mixture in the skillet. Cook for 2-3 minutes, or until heated through.
6. Add cooked pasta to the skillet and toss to coat.
7. Serve hot, garnished with fresh basil.

60. VEGAN JACKFRUIT TACOS

Ingredients:
- 1 can (20 oz) young green jackfruit in brine, drained and rinsed
- 1 tablespoon olive oil
- 1 onion, chopped
- 2 cloves garlic, minced
- 1 bell pepper, chopped
- 1 teaspoon ground cumin
- 1 teaspoon chili powder
- 1/2 teaspoon smoked paprika

- Salt and pepper, to taste
- 1/2 cup vegetable broth
- 8 small corn tortillas
- Toppings: avocado, salsa, cilantro, lime wedges

Instructions:
1. Shred the jackfruit using your hands or a fork.
2. In a large skillet, heat olive oil over medium heat. Add onion and garlic. Cook until softened, about 5 minutes.
3. Stir in bell pepper, shredded jackfruit, cumin, chili powder, smoked paprika, salt, and pepper. Cook for another 5 minutes.
4. Add vegetable broth to the skillet. Bring to a simmer and cook for 10-15 minutes, or until jackfruit is tender and broth has been absorbed.
5. Warm corn tortillas in a dry skillet or microwave.
6. To assemble the tacos, fill each tortilla with the jackfruit mixture. Top with avocado, salsa, cilantro, and a squeeze of lime juice.
7. Serve hot.

61. VEGAN CAULIFLOWER ALFREDO

Ingredients:
- 8 oz fettuccine pasta
- 1 small head cauliflower, chopped
- 2 tablespoons olive oil
- 2 cloves garlic, minced
- 1/2 cup vegetable broth
- 1/2 cup unsweetened almond milk
- 1/4 cup nutritional yeast
- 1 tablespoon lemon juice
- Salt and pepper, to taste
- Fresh parsley, for garnish

Instructions:
1. Cook fettuccine pasta according to package instructions. Drain and set aside.

2. Steam chopped cauliflower until tender, about 10-15 minutes. Drain and set aside.

3. In a large skillet, heat olive oil over medium heat. Add garlic and cook for 1 minute, or until fragrant.

4. Add steamed cauliflower, vegetable broth, almond milk, nutritional yeast, lemon juice, salt, and pepper to the skillet.

5. Using an immersion blender or regular blender, blend until smooth and creamy.

6. Add cooked pasta to the skillet and toss to coat.

7. Serve hot, garnished with fresh parsley.

62. VEGAN MUSHROOM STROGANOFF

Ingredients:
- 8 oz pasta of choice
- 2 tablespoons olive oil
- 1 onion, chopped
- 2 cloves garlic, minced
- 8 oz mushrooms, sliced
- 1 can (15 oz) white beans, drained and rinsed
- 1 cup vegetable broth
- 1 tablespoon soy sauce
- 1/2 cup vegan sour cream
- Salt and pepper, to taste
- Fresh parsley, for garnish

Instructions:
1. Cook pasta according to package instructions. Drain and set aside.

2. In a large skillet, heat olive oil over medium heat. Add onion and garlic. Cook until softened, about 5 minutes.

3. Add mushrooms and cook for another 5 minutes, or until mushrooms are tender.

4. Stir in white beans, vegetable broth, and soy sauce. Simmer for 10 minutes.

5. Remove from heat and stir in vegan sour cream. Season with salt and pepper.

6. Serve over cooked pasta, garnished with fresh parsley.

63. VEGAN LENTIL SHEPHERD'S PIE

Ingredients:
- 1 cup green lentils, rinsed and drained
- 2 cups vegetable broth
- 1 onion, chopped
- 2 carrots, diced
- 2 celery stalks, diced
- 2 cloves garlic, minced
- 1 teaspoon dried thyme
- 1 teaspoon dried rosemary
- Salt and pepper, to taste
- 4 cups mashed potatoes

Instructions:
1. Preheat the oven to 400°F (200°C).

2. In a large pot, combine lentils and vegetable broth. Bring to a boil, then reduce heat and simmer for 20-25 minutes, or until lentils are tender.

3. In a skillet, heat olive oil over medium heat. Add onion, carrots, celery, and garlic. Sauté for 5-7 minutes, or until vegetables are softened.

4. Add cooked lentils, thyme, rosemary, salt, and pepper to the skillet. Cook for another 5 minutes.

5. Spoon the lentil mixture into a baking dish.

6. Spread mashed potatoes over the lentil mixture.

7. Bake for 20-25 minutes, or until the mashed potatoes are lightly browned.

8. Serve hot.

64. VEGAN LEMON ASPARAGUS PASTA

Ingredients:
- 8 oz spaghetti

- 1 bunch asparagus, trimmed and cut into 2-inch pieces
- 2 tablespoons olive oil
- 2 cloves garlic, minced
- Zest and juice of 1 lemon
- 1/4 cup chopped fresh parsley
- Salt and pepper, to taste

Instructions:
1. Cook spaghetti according to package instructions. Drain and set aside.
2. In a large skillet, heat olive oil over medium heat. Add garlic and cook for 1 minute, or until fragrant.
3. Add asparagus to the skillet. Cook for 5-7 minutes, or until tender-crisp.
4. Stir in cooked spaghetti, lemon zest, lemon juice, parsley, salt, and pepper. Cook for another 2-3 minutes, or until heated through.
5. Serve hot.

65. VEGAN THAI GREEN CURRY

Ingredients:
- 1 tablespoon olive oil
- 1 onion, chopped
- 2 cloves garlic, minced
- 2 tablespoons green curry paste
- 1 can (14 oz) coconut milk
- 1 cup vegetable broth
- 1 bell pepper, sliced
- 1 zucchini, sliced
- 1 cup sliced mushrooms
- 1 cup chopped broccoli
- 1 can (15 oz) chickpeas, drained and rinsed
- Salt and pepper, to taste
- Cooked rice, for serving
- Fresh cilantro, for garnish

Instructions:

1. Heat olive oil in a large pot over medium heat. Add onion and garlic. Cook until softened, about 5 minutes.
2. Stir in green curry paste and cook for another 2 minutes.
3. Add coconut milk and vegetable broth to the pot. Bring to a simmer.
4. Add bell pepper, zucchini, mushrooms, broccoli, and

Chapter 4: Snack and Side Dish Recipes

66. SPICY ROASTED CHICKPEAS

Ingredients:
- 1 can (15 oz) chickpeas, drained and rinsed
- 1 tablespoon olive oil
- 1 teaspoon paprika
- 1/2 teaspoon cayenne pepper
- 1/2 teaspoon garlic powder
- Salt, to taste

Instructions:
1. Preheat the oven to 400°F (200°C).
2. Pat the chickpeas dry with a paper towel.
3. In a bowl, toss the chickpeas with olive oil, paprika, cayenne pepper, garlic powder, and salt.
4. Spread the chickpeas on a baking sheet in a single layer.
5. Roast in the oven for 25-30 minutes, or until crispy.
6. Let cool before serving.

67. AVOCADO HUMMUS

Ingredients:
- 1 can (15 oz) chickpeas, drained and rinsed
- 1 ripe avocado, peeled and pitted
- 2 tablespoons tahini
- 2 tablespoons lemon juice
- 1 clove garlic, minced
- 1/2 teaspoon cumin
- Salt and pepper, to taste

Instructions:
1. In a food processor, combine chickpeas, avocado, tahini, lemon juice, garlic, cumin, salt, and pepper.

2. Blend until smooth and creamy.
3. Serve with vegetables or pita chips.

68. VEGAN SPINACH AND ARTICHOKE DIP

Ingredients:
- 1 can (14 oz) artichoke hearts, drained and chopped
- 1 cup frozen chopped spinach, thawed and drained
- 1/2 cup vegan mayonnaise
- 1/2 cup vegan cream cheese
- 1/4 cup nutritional yeast
- 1/4 cup chopped green onions
- 1 clove garlic, minced
- Salt and pepper, to taste

Instructions:
1. Preheat the oven to 350°F (175°C).
2. In a bowl, combine artichoke hearts, spinach, vegan mayonnaise, vegan cream cheese, nutritional yeast, green onions, garlic, salt, and pepper.
3. Transfer the mixture to a baking dish.
4. Bake for 20-25 minutes, or until bubbly and golden.
5. Serve hot with crackers or bread.

69. VEGAN GARLIC MASHED POTATOES

Ingredients:
- 2 lbs Yukon Gold potatoes, peeled and diced
- 4 cloves garlic, minced
- 1/2 cup unsweetened almond milk
- 2 tablespoons vegan butter
- Salt and pepper, to taste
- Chopped chives, for garnish

Instructions:
1. Place diced potatoes and minced garlic in a large pot. Cover with water and bring to a boil.
2. Reduce heat and simmer for 15-20 minutes, or until potatoes are tender.
3. Drain the potatoes and garlic, reserving 1/4 cup of the cooking water.
4. Mash the potatoes and garlic with a potato masher.
5. Stir in almond milk, vegan butter, salt, pepper, and reserved cooking water until smooth and creamy.
6. Serve hot, garnished with chopped chives.

70. ROASTED VEGETABLES

Ingredients:
- Assorted vegetables (e.g., carrots, bell peppers, zucchini, onions, cherry tomatoes)
- Olive oil
- Salt and pepper, to taste
- Fresh herbs (e.g., rosemary, thyme), chopped

Instructions:
1. Preheat the oven to 400°F (200°C).
2. Chop vegetables into bite-sized pieces.
3. Toss vegetables with olive oil, salt, pepper, and fresh herbs.
4. Spread vegetables in a single layer on a baking sheet.
5. Roast in the oven for 20-25 minutes, or until vegetables are tender and slightly caramelized.
6. Serve hot.

71. VEGAN BUFFALO CAULIFLOWER WINGS

Ingredients:
- 1 head cauliflower, cut into florets
- 1/2 cup all-purpose flour
- 1/2 cup unsweetened almond milk
- 1 teaspoon garlic powder

- 1 teaspoon onion powder
- 1/2 teaspoon smoked paprika
- Salt and pepper, to taste
- 1/2 cup hot sauce
- 2 tablespoons vegan butter, melted

Instructions:
1. Preheat the oven to 450°F (230°C).
2. In a bowl, whisk together flour, almond milk, garlic powder, onion powder, smoked paprika, salt, and pepper.
3. Dip cauliflower florets into the batter, shaking off excess.
4. Place cauliflower on a baking sheet lined with parchment paper.
5. Bake for 20-25 minutes, or until the cauliflower is tender and the batter is crispy.
6. In a separate bowl, combine hot sauce and melted vegan butter.
7. Toss baked cauliflower in the hot sauce mixture until coated.
8. Serve hot with vegan ranch dressing and celery sticks.

72. VEGAN ZUCCHINI CHIPS

Ingredients:
- 2 zucchinis, thinly sliced
- 2 tablespoons olive oil
- 1/4 cup nutritional yeast
- 1 teaspoon garlic powder
- 1 teaspoon onion powder
- 1/2 teaspoon paprika
- Salt and pepper, to taste

Instructions:
1. Preheat the oven to 425°F (220°C).
2. Place zucchini slices in a single layer on a baking sheet lined with parchment paper.
3. Drizzle olive oil over the zucchini slices.

4. In a small bowl, combine nutritional yeast, garlic powder, onion powder, paprika, salt, and pepper.
5. Sprinkle the nutritional yeast mixture over the zucchini slices.
6. Bake for 15-20 minutes, or until zucchini chips are crispy.
7. Let cool before serving.

73. VEGAN QUINOA TABBOULEH

Ingredients:
- 1 cup quinoa, cooked and cooled
- 1 cucumber, diced
- 2 tomatoes, diced
- 1/2 red onion, finely chopped
- 1/4 cup chopped fresh parsley
- 1/4 cup chopped fresh mint
- 1/4 cup lemon juice
- 2 tablespoons olive oil
- Salt and pepper, to taste

Instructions:
1. In a large bowl, combine quinoa, cucumber, tomatoes, red onion, parsley, and mint.
2. In a small bowl, whisk together lemon juice, olive oil, salt, and pepper.
3. Pour the dressing over the quinoa mixture and toss to combine.
4. Serve chilled.

74. VEGAN CAULIFLOWER RICE

Ingredients:
- 1 head cauliflower, grated
- 2 tablespoons olive oil
- 2 cloves garlic, minced
- 1/2 teaspoon cumin
- 1/2 teaspoon smoked paprika
- Salt and pepper, to taste

- Fresh cilantro, for garnish

Instructions:
1. In a large skillet, heat olive oil over medium heat. Add garlic and cook for 1 minute, or until fragrant.
2. Add grated cauliflower to the skillet. Cook for 5-7 minutes, or until cauliflower is tender.
3. Stir in cumin, smoked paprika, salt, and pepper.
4. Cook for another 2-3 minutes, or until heated through.
5. Serve hot, garnished with fresh cilantro.

75. VEGAN CAPRESE SALAD

Ingredients:
- 2 large tomatoes, sliced
- 1 package (8 oz) vegan mozzarella cheese, sliced
- 1/4 cup fresh basil leaves
- 2 tablespoons balsamic glaze
- Salt and pepper, to taste

Instructions:
1. Arrange tomato slices and vegan mozzarella slices on a serving platter.
2. Tuck fresh basil leaves between the tomato and mozzarella slices.
3. Drizzle balsamic glaze over the salad.
4. Season with salt and pepper.
5. Serve chilled.

76. VEGAN SPINACH ARTICHOKE DIP

Ingredients:
- 1 can (14 oz) artichoke hearts, drained and chopped
- 1 cup frozen chopped spinach, thawed and drained
- 1 cup vegan mayonnaise
- 1 cup vegan cream cheese
- 1/2 cup nutritional yeast

- 1/4 cup chopped green onions
- 2 cloves garlic, minced
- Salt and pepper, to taste

Instructions:
1. Preheat the oven to 350°F (175°C).
2. In a bowl, combine artichoke hearts, spinach, vegan mayonnaise, vegan cream cheese, nutritional yeast, green onions, garlic, salt, and pepper.
3. Transfer the mixture to a baking dish.
4. Bake for 20-25 minutes, or until bubbly and golden.
5. Serve hot with crackers or bread.

77. VEGAN STUFFED MUSHROOMS

Ingredients:
- 12 large mushrooms, stems removed
- 1/2 cup vegan cream cheese
- 1/4 cup nutritional yeast
- 2 tablespoons chopped fresh parsley
- 2 cloves garlic, minced
- Salt and pepper, to taste
- Olive oil, for drizzling

Instructions:
1. Preheat the oven to 375°F (190°C).
2. In a bowl, combine vegan cream cheese, nutritional yeast, parsley, garlic, salt, and pepper.
3. Spoon the mixture into the mushroom caps.
4. Place stuffed mushrooms on a baking sheet.
5. Drizzle with olive oil.
6. Bake for 15-20 minutes, or until mushrooms are tender.
7. Serve hot.

78. VEGAN COLESLAW

Ingredients:
- 4 cups shredded cabbage
- 1 carrot, grated
- 1/2 cup vegan mayonnaise
- 2 tablespoons apple cider vinegar
- 1 tablespoon maple syrup
- 1 teaspoon Dijon mustard
- Salt and pepper, to taste

Instructions:
1. In a large bowl, combine shredded cabbage and grated carrot.
2. In a small bowl, whisk together vegan mayonnaise, apple cider vinegar, maple syrup, Dijon mustard, salt, and pepper.
3. Pour the dressing over the cabbage mixture.
4. Toss to combine.
5. Refrigerate for at least 1 hour before serving.

79. VEGAN ROASTED BRUSSELS SPROUTS

Ingredients:
- 1 lb Brussels sprouts, trimmed and halved
- 2 tablespoons olive oil
- 2 tablespoons balsamic vinegar
- 2 cloves garlic, minced
- Salt and pepper, to taste

Instructions:
1. Preheat the oven to 400°F (200°C).
2. In a bowl, toss Brussels sprouts with olive oil, balsamic vinegar, garlic, salt, and pepper.
3. Spread Brussels sprouts in a single layer on a baking sheet.
4. Roast in the oven for 25-30 minutes, or until Brussels sprouts are tender and caramelized.
5. Serve hot.

80. VEGAN SMASHED POTATOES

Ingredients:
- 1 lb baby potatoes
- 2 tablespoons olive oil
- 2 cloves garlic, minced
- 1/4 cup chopped fresh parsley
- Salt and pepper, to taste

Instructions:
1. Place baby potatoes in a pot and cover with water.
2. Bring to a boil, then reduce heat and simmer for 15-20 minutes, or until potatoes are tender.
3. Drain the potatoes and let cool slightly.
4. Preheat the oven to 425°F (220°C).
5. Place potatoes on a baking sheet and gently smash with a fork.
6. Drizzle olive oil over the smashed potatoes.
7. Sprinkle with garlic, parsley, salt, and pepper.
8. Roast in the oven for 20-25 minutes, or until potatoes are crispy.
9. Serve hot.

81. VEGAN SWEET POTATO FRIES

Ingredients:
- 2 large sweet potatoes, peeled and cut into fries
- 2 tablespoons olive oil
- 1 teaspoon smoked paprika
- 1/2 teaspoon garlic powder
- 1/2 teaspoon onion powder
- Salt and pepper, to taste

Instructions:

1. Preheat the oven to 425°F (220°C).

2. In a bowl, toss sweet potato fries with olive oil, smoked paprika, garlic powder, onion powder, salt, and pepper.

3. Spread fries in a single layer on a baking sheet lined with parchment paper.

4. Bake for 20-25 minutes, flipping halfway through, or until fries are crispy.

5. Serve hot.

82. VEGAN PUMPKIN SEED CRUNCH

Ingredients:
- 1 cup raw pumpkin seeds
- 1 tablespoon olive oil
- 1 teaspoon smoked paprika
- 1/2 teaspoon garlic powder
- 1/2 teaspoon onion powder
- Salt, to taste

Instructions:
1. Preheat the oven to 300°F (150°C).

2. In a bowl, toss pumpkin seeds with olive oil, smoked paprika, garlic powder, onion powder, and salt.

3. Spread pumpkin seeds in a single layer on a baking sheet lined with parchment paper.

4. Bake for 20-25 minutes, stirring halfway through, or until pumpkin seeds are crispy.

5. Let cool before serving.

83. VEGAN CREAMY MASHED CAULIFLOWER

Ingredients:
- 1 head cauliflower, chopped
- 2 tablespoons vegan cream cheese

- 2 tablespoons nutritional yeast
- 1 clove garlic, minced
- Salt and pepper, to taste
- Chopped chives, for garnish

Instructions:
1. Steam cauliflower until tender, about 10-15 minutes.
2. In a bowl, combine steamed cauliflower, vegan cream cheese, nutritional yeast, garlic, salt, and pepper.
3. Use a potato masher or immersion blender to mash the cauliflower until smooth and creamy.
4. Serve hot, garnished with chopped chives.

84. VEGAN MAPLE ROASTED CARROTS

Ingredients:
- 1 lb carrots, peeled and sliced into sticks
- 2 tablespoons olive oil
- 2 tablespoons maple syrup
- 1/2 teaspoon cinnamon
- Salt and pepper, to taste

Instructions:
1. Preheat the oven to 400°F (200°C).
2. In a bowl, toss carrot sticks with olive oil, maple syrup, cinnamon, salt, and pepper.
3. Spread carrots in a single layer on a baking sheet lined with parchment paper.
4. Roast in the oven for 20-25 minutes, or until carrots are tender and caramelized.
5. Serve hot.

85. VEGAN LEMON GARLIC GREEN BEANS

Ingredients:

- 1 lb green beans, trimmed
- 2 tablespoons olive oil
- 2 cloves garlic, minced
- Zest and juice of 1 lemon
- Salt and pepper, to taste

 Instructions:
1. In a large skillet, heat olive oil over medium heat. Add garlic and cook for 1 minute, or until fragrant.
2. Add green beans to the skillet. Cook for 5-7 minutes, or until beans are tender-crisp.
3. Stir in lemon zest, lemon juice, salt, and pepper.
4. Cook for another 2-3 minutes, or until heated through.
5. Serve hot.

Chapter 5: Dessert Recipes

86. VEGAN CHOCOLATE AVOCADO MOUSSE

Ingredients:
- 2 ripe avocados, peeled and pitted
- 1/2 cup cocoa powder
- 1/2 cup maple syrup
- 1 teaspoon vanilla extract
- Pinch of salt
- Vegan whipped cream, for serving (optional)

Instructions:
1. In a food processor, blend avocados, cocoa powder, maple syrup, vanilla extract, and salt until smooth and creamy.
2. Divide the mousse into serving cups.
3. Refrigerate for at least 30 minutes before serving.
4. Serve chilled, topped with vegan whipped cream if desired.

87. VEGAN BANANA BREAD

Ingredients:
- 3 ripe bananas, mashed
- 1/3 cup melted coconut oil
- 1/2 cup maple syrup
- 1/4 cup almond milk
- 1 teaspoon vanilla extract
- 1 3/4 cups whole wheat flour
- 1 teaspoon baking soda
- 1/2 teaspoon salt
- 1/2 cup chopped walnuts (optional)

Instructions:
1. Preheat the oven to 325°F (165°C). Grease a 9x5-inch loaf pan.

2. In a large bowl, combine mashed bananas, coconut oil, maple syrup, almond milk, and vanilla extract.
3. Add flour, baking soda, and salt. Stir until just combined. Fold in chopped walnuts, if using.
4. Pour the batter into the prepared loaf pan.
5. Bake for 60-65 minutes, or until a toothpick inserted into the center comes out clean.
6. Let cool before slicing.

88. VEGAN BLUEBERRY COCONUT PARFAIT

Ingredients:
- 1 can (13.5 oz) full-fat coconut milk, refrigerated overnight
- 1 tablespoon maple syrup
- 1/2 teaspoon vanilla extract
- 1 cup fresh blueberries
- 1/4 cup shredded coconut, toasted

Instructions:
1. Open the can of coconut milk and scoop out the solid coconut cream that has risen to the top. Discard the liquid or save it for another use.
2. In a bowl, whisk together coconut cream, maple syrup, and vanilla extract until smooth.
3. In serving glasses, layer coconut cream, blueberries, and toasted coconut.
4. Repeat layers until glasses are filled.
5. Serve immediately or refrigerate until ready to serve.

89. VEGAN CHOCOLATE CHIP COOKIES

Ingredients:
- 1/2 cup coconut oil, melted
- 1/2 cup maple syrup
- 1 teaspoon vanilla extract
- 2 cups almond flour
- 1/2 teaspoon baking soda

- 1/2 teaspoon salt
- 1/2 cup vegan chocolate chips

Instructions:
1. Preheat the oven to 350°F (175°C). Line a baking sheet with parchment paper.
2. In a bowl, whisk together melted coconut oil, maple syrup, and vanilla extract.
3. Add almond flour, baking soda, and salt. Stir until well combined.
4. Fold in vegan chocolate chips.
5. Drop spoonfuls of dough onto the prepared baking sheet.
6. Bake for 10-12 minutes, or until the edges are golden brown.
7. Let cool on the baking sheet for 5 minutes before transferring to a wire rack to cool completely.

90. VEGAN APPLE CRISP

Ingredients:
- 4 cups apples, peeled, cored, and sliced
- 1 tablespoon lemon juice
- 1/4 cup maple syrup
- 1 teaspoon cinnamon
- 1/2 cup rolled oats
- 1/4 cup almond flour
- 1/4 cup chopped nuts (such as pecans or walnuts)
- 2 tablespoons coconut oil, melted
- 2 tablespoons maple syrup

Instructions:
1. Preheat the oven to 350°F (175°C). Grease a baking dish.
2. In a bowl, toss apples with lemon juice, maple syrup, and cinnamon. Spread evenly in the prepared baking dish.
3. In another bowl, combine rolled oats, almond flour, chopped nuts, melted coconut oil, and maple syrup. Mix until crumbly.
4. Sprinkle the oat mixture over the apples.

5. Bake for 30-35 minutes, or until the topping is golden brown and the apples are tender.
6. Serve warm, optionally with vegan ice cream or whipped cream.

91. VEGAN CHOCOLATE TRUFFLES

Ingredients:
- 1/2 cup coconut cream
- 8 oz dairy-free dark chocolate, chopped
- 1 teaspoon vanilla extract
- Cocoa powder, for rolling (optional)

Instructions:
1. In a saucepan, heat coconut cream until simmering.
2. Remove from heat and add chopped dark chocolate. Let sit for 2-3 minutes, then stir until smooth.
3. Stir in vanilla extract.
4. Refrigerate the mixture for 2 hours, or until firm.
5. Using a spoon, scoop out small portions of the mixture and roll into balls.
6. Roll the truffles in cocoa powder, if desired.
7. Store in the refrigerator until ready to serve.

92. VEGAN RASPBERRY CHEESECAKE BARS

Ingredients:
- 1 1/2 cups almond flour
- 1/4 cup coconut oil, melted
- 1/4 cup maple syrup
- 1 can (14 oz) coconut cream, refrigerated overnight
- 1/4 cup powdered sugar
- 1 teaspoon vanilla extract
- 1 cup fresh raspberries

Instructions:

1. Preheat the oven to 350°F (175°C). Line a baking dish with parchment paper.
2. In a bowl, combine almond flour, melted coconut oil, and maple syrup. Press into the bottom of the prepared baking dish.
3. Bake for 10-12 minutes, or until lightly golden. Let cool.
4. In a bowl, beat coconut cream, powdered sugar, and vanilla extract until smooth.
5. Spread the coconut cream mixture over the cooled crust.
6. Top with fresh raspberries.
7. Refrigerate for at least 1 hour before slicing into bars.

93. VEGAN PEANUT BUTTER COOKIES

Ingredients:
- 1/2 cup coconut oil, melted
- 1/2 cup peanut butter
- 1/2 cup coconut sugar
- 1/4 cup maple syrup
- 1 teaspoon vanilla extract
- 1 1/2 cups oat flour
- 1/2 teaspoon baking soda
- 1/4 teaspoon salt
- Vegan chocolate chips, for topping (optional)

Instructions:
1. Preheat the oven to 350°F (175°C). Line a baking sheet with parchment paper.
2. In a bowl, combine melted coconut oil, peanut butter, coconut sugar, maple syrup, and vanilla extract.
3. Add oat flour, baking soda, and salt. Mix until well combined.
4. Roll the dough into balls and place them on the prepared baking sheet.
5. Flatten the balls with a fork to create a crisscross pattern. Optionally, top with vegan chocolate chips.
6. Bake for 10-12 minutes, or until golden brown.

7. Let cool on the baking sheet for 5 minutes before transferring to a wire
rack to cool completely.

94. VEGAN LEMON BARS

Ingredients:
- 1 1/2 cups almond flour
- 1/4 cup coconut oil, melted
- 1/4 cup maple syrup
- 1 can (14 oz) full-fat coconut milk, refrigerated overnight
- 1/2 cup lemon juice
- 1/2 cup maple syrup
- 2 tablespoons cornstarch
- Zest of 1 lemon
- Powdered sugar, for dusting (optional)

Instructions:
1. Preheat the oven to 350°F (175°C). Line a baking dish with parchment
paper.
2. In a bowl, combine almond flour, melted coconut oil, and maple syrup.
Press into the bottom of the prepared baking dish.
3. Bake for 10-12 minutes, or until lightly golden. Let cool.
4. In a saucepan, combine the thick coconut cream (scooped from the top of
the refrigerated can), lemon juice, maple syrup, cornstarch, and lemon zest.
Cook over medium heat, stirring constantly, until thickened.
5. Pour the lemon mixture over the cooled crust. Spread evenly.
6. Refrigerate for at least 2 hours, or until set.
7. Dust with powdered sugar before serving, if desired.

95. VEGAN CHERRY ALMOND CRISP

Ingredients:
- 4 cups cherries, pitted
- 1 tablespoon lemon juice

- 1/4 cup maple syrup
- 1 teaspoon almond extract
- 1 cup rolled oats
- 1/2 cup almond flour
- 1/4 cup coconut sugar
- 1/4 cup sliced almonds
- 1/4 cup coconut oil, melted
- Pinch of salt

 Instructions:
1. Preheat the oven to 350°F (175°C). Grease a baking dish.
2. In a bowl, combine cherries, lemon juice, maple syrup, and almond extract. Spread evenly in the prepared baking dish.
3. In another bowl, combine rolled oats, almond flour, coconut sugar, sliced almonds, melted coconut oil, and salt. Mix until crumbly.
4. Sprinkle the oat mixture over the cherries.
5. Bake for 30-35 minutes, or until the topping is golden brown and the cherries are bubbly.
6. Serve warm, optionally with vegan ice cream.

96. VEGAN COCONUT MACAROONS

 Ingredients:
- 2 1/2 cups shredded coconut
- 1/2 cup almond flour
- 1/2 cup maple syrup
- 1/4 cup coconut oil, melted
- 1 teaspoon vanilla extract
- Pinch of salt
- Vegan chocolate, melted (optional)

 Instructions:
1. Preheat the oven to 350°F (175°C). Line a baking sheet with parchment paper.

2. In a bowl, combine shredded coconut, almond flour, maple syrup, melted coconut oil, vanilla extract, and salt. Mix until well combined.
3. Scoop tablespoon-sized mounds of the mixture onto the prepared baking sheet.
4. Bake for 15-20 minutes, or until golden brown.
5. Let cool completely on the baking sheet.
6. Optionally, dip the cooled macaroons in melted vegan chocolate.
7. Let the chocolate set before serving.

97. VEGAN PUMPKIN PIE

Ingredients:
- 1 1/2 cups pumpkin puree
- 1/2 cup coconut milk
- 1/2 cup maple syrup
- 2 tablespoons cornstarch
- 1 teaspoon vanilla extract
- 1 teaspoon cinnamon
- 1/2 teaspoon ground ginger
- 1/4 teaspoon ground nutmeg
- 1/4 teaspoon ground cloves
- 1/4 teaspoon salt
- 1 prepared vegan pie crust

Instructions:
1. Preheat the oven to 350°F (175°C).
2. In a bowl, whisk together pumpkin puree, coconut milk, maple syrup, cornstarch, vanilla extract, cinnamon, ginger, nutmeg, cloves, and salt until smooth.
3. Pour the pumpkin mixture into the prepared pie crust.
4. Bake for 50-60 minutes, or until the filling is set.
5. Let cool completely before slicing and serving.

Chapter 6: Drinks

98. VEGAN STRAWBERRY COCONUT SMOOTHIE

Ingredients:
- 1 cup coconut milk
- 1 cup fresh or frozen strawberries
- 1 banana
- 1 tablespoon maple syrup
- 1/2 teaspoon vanilla extract

Instructions:
1. Blend all ingredients in a blender until smooth.
2. Serve immediately.

99. VEGAN GOLDEN MILK

Ingredients:
- 1 cup almond milk
- 1 teaspoon ground turmeric
- 1/2 teaspoon ground cinnamon
- 1/4 teaspoon ground ginger
- Pinch of black pepper
- 1 teaspoon maple syrup

Instructions:
1. In a small saucepan, heat almond milk over medium heat until warm but not boiling.
2. Whisk in turmeric, cinnamon, ginger, black pepper, and maple syrup.
3. Continue to heat for another minute, stirring constantly.
4. Remove from heat and strain if desired.
5. Serve warm.

100. VEGAN ICED MATCHA LATTE

Ingredients:
- 1 teaspoon matcha powder
- 1 tablespoon hot water
- 1 cup almond milk
- 1 tablespoon maple syrup
- Ice cubes

Instructions:
1. In a glass, whisk matcha powder with hot water until smooth.
2. Add almond milk and maple syrup. Stir to combine.
3. Fill the glass with ice cubes.
4. Serve cold.

101. VEGAN WATERMELON AGUA FRESCA

Ingredients:
- 4 cups cubed watermelon
- 2 cups water
- 1 tablespoon lime juice
- 1-2 tablespoons agave syrup, to taste
- Ice cubes
- Fresh mint leaves, for garnish

Instructions:
1. In a blender, blend watermelon, water, lime juice, and agave syrup until smooth.
2. Strain the mixture if desired.
3. Serve over ice cubes, garnished with fresh mint leaves.

102. VEGAN SPICED CHAI TEA LATTE

Ingredients:
- 1 cup almond milk
- 1 black tea bag
- 1/2 teaspoon ground cinnamon

- 1/4 teaspoon ground ginger
- 1/8 teaspoon ground cloves
- 1/8 teaspoon ground cardamom
- 1 tablespoon maple syrup

Instructions:
1. In a small saucepan, heat almond milk over medium heat until warm but not boiling.
2. Add the tea bag and let steep for 3-5 minutes.
3. Remove the tea bag and whisk in cinnamon, ginger, cloves, cardamom, and maple syrup.
4. Continue to heat for another minute, stirring constantly.
5. Remove from heat and strain if desired.
6. Serve warm.

103. VEGAN LAVENDER LEMONADE

Ingredients:
- 1/2 cup fresh lemon juice
- 4 cups water
- 1/2 cup agave syrup
- 1 tablespoon dried lavender buds
- Ice cubes
- Fresh lavender sprigs, for garnish

Instructions:
1. In a small saucepan, combine water, agave syrup, and dried lavender buds.
2. Bring to a simmer over medium heat, then remove from heat and let steep for 15-20 minutes.
3. Strain the lavender syrup and let cool.
4. In a pitcher, combine fresh lemon juice, lavender syrup, and water.
5. Stir to combine.
6. Serve over ice cubes, garnished with fresh lavender sprigs.

104. VEGAN MANGO LASSI

Ingredients:
- 1 cup diced mango
- 1/2 cup coconut yogurt
- 1/2 cup almond milk
- 1 tablespoon maple syrup
- 1/2 teaspoon ground cardamom
- Ice cubes

Instructions:
1. In a blender, combine diced mango, coconut yogurt, almond milk, maple syrup, and ground cardamom.
2. Blend until smooth.
3. Serve over ice cubes.

105. VEGAN MINT MOJITO

Ingredients:
- 1/4 cup fresh mint leaves
- 2 tablespoons lime juice
- 1 tablespoon agave syrup
- 1/2 cup sparkling water
- Ice cubes
- Lime slices, for garnish

Instructions:
1. In a glass, muddle mint leaves with lime juice and agave syrup.
2. Fill the glass with ice cubes.
3. Top with sparkling water.
4. Stir to combine.
5. Garnish with lime slices.

106. VEGAN ICED COFFEE

Ingredients:
- 1 cup cold brewed coffee
- 1/2 cup almond milk
- 1 tablespoon maple syrup
- Ice cubes

Instructions:
1. In a glass, combine cold brewed coffee, almond milk, and maple syrup.
2. Stir to combine.
3. Fill the glass with ice cubes.
4. Serve cold.

107. VEGAN PEACH SMOOTHIE

Ingredients:
- 1 cup sliced peaches (fresh or frozen)
- 1 banana
- 1/2 cup coconut milk
- 1/2 cup orange juice
- 1 tablespoon maple syrup
- Ice cubes

Instructions:
1. In a blender, combine sliced peaches, banana, coconut milk, orange juice, and maple syrup.
2. Blend until smooth.
3. Serve cold.

108. VEGAN CUCUMBER MINT COOLER

Ingredients:
- 1 cucumber, peeled and chopped
- 1/4 cup fresh mint leaves

- 2 tablespoons lime juice
- 2 tablespoons agave syrup
- 2 cups water
- Ice cubes

Instructions:
1. In a blender, combine chopped cucumber, mint leaves, lime juice, agave syrup, and water.
2. Blend until smooth.
3. Strain the mixture if desired.
4. Serve over ice cubes.

109. VEGAN ORANGE CREAMSICLE SMOOTHIE

Ingredients:
- 1 cup orange juice
- 1/2 cup coconut milk
- 1/2 teaspoon vanilla extract
- 1 tablespoon agave syrup
- Ice cubes

Instructions:
1. In a blender, combine orange juice, coconut milk, vanilla extract, and agave syrup.
2. Blend until smooth.
3. Serve cold.

110. VEGAN PINEAPPLE GINGER COOLER

Ingredients:
- 2 cups pineapple chunks
- 1-inch piece of ginger, peeled and chopped
- 2 tablespoons lime juice
- 2 tablespoons agave syrup
- 2 cups water

- Ice cubes
- Pineapple slices and mint leaves, for garnish

Instructions:
1. In a blender, combine pineapple chunks, chopped ginger, lime juice, agave syrup, and water.
2. Blend until smooth.
3. Strain the mixture if desired.
4. Serve over ice cubes, garnished with pineapple slices and mint leaves.

Conclusion

As we reach the end of "Plant-Based Lupus Cookbook for Women," I hope this collection of recipes has provided you with nourishing and delicious options to support your health and well-being. Living with lupus can present challenges, but focusing on a plant-based diet rich in nutrients and antioxidants can help manage symptoms and promote overall wellness.

Each recipe in this book has been thoughtfully crafted to be flavorful, satisfying, and easy to prepare. Whether you're looking for hearty meals, comforting soups, or indulgent desserts, there's something here for every craving and occasion.

Remember, cooking is a form of self-care. Taking the time to prepare wholesome meals not only benefits your body but also nourishes your soul. Embrace the joy of cooking and savor each bite, knowing that you're nourishing your body with the best nature has to offer.

I hope these recipes inspire you to get creative in the kitchen and discover new ways to enjoy plant-based eating. May your journey to health and wellness be filled with delicious food and joyful moments shared with loved ones.

Thank you for choosing "Plant-Based Lupus Cookbook for Women." Here's to good health and happy cooking!